# MIND DIET COOKBOOK FOR SENIORS

A Comprehensive Guide To 50 Wholesome Recipes for Alzheimer's, Dementia, and Cognitive Enhancement | 7-Day Meal Plan Included

Corey Pearce

## OTHER BOOKS BY THIS AUTHOR

# Table of Contents

# Introduction

In the calm refuge of your sunny house, you, a vibrant senior, hold the key to a brighter, more nimble mind. Your quest starts when you find the "Mind Diet Cookbook for Seniors."

With curiosity and a thirst for greater mental abilities, you go on an excursion through the cookbook's pages. The delectable meals contain an assortment of "Mind foods" — vivid leafy greens, sweet berries, heart-healthy fish, and tasty almonds. These components claim to boost your memory and cognitive performance.

As you explore the recipes, you discover delight in making and eating these wonderful meals that nourish your brain. The Mediterranean-inspired meals and the taste of healthy, nutrient-rich ingredients enchant your senses. You gladly share your newfound culinary discoveries with friends and family, stimulating exciting discussions over shared meals.

The findings amaze you. Over time, your memory and mental clarity increase. You feel more alert, concentrated, and full of life. Your cognitive well-being develops, and you enjoy your senior years with the passion of someone far younger.

The "Mind Diet Cookbook for Seniors" is more than just a cookbook; it's your valued companion on your road to greater brain health, a reminder that age is only a number when you nourish your mind with care and taste.

# Chapter 1: Understanding the Mind Diet

The Mind Diet is not merely a diet; it's a lifestyle approach to eating that prioritizes foods proven to enhance brain health. It's a fusion of two well-respected diets: the Mediterranean Diet and the DASH (Dietary Approaches to Stop Hypertension) Diet.

By combining the strengths of these diets, the Mind Diet emphasizes the consumption of nutrient-rich, whole foods, particularly fruits, vegetables, whole grains, fish, and nuts.

These ingredients have been associated with improved cognitive function and reduced risk of conditions like Alzheimer's disease.

## Benefits of the Mind Diet for Seniors

For seniors, embracing the Mind Diet brings numerous advantages. It offers the promise of maintaining mental clarity, enhancing memory, and reducing the risk of cognitive disorders. Additionally, the Mind Diet promotes overall well-being, as many of its core principles align with heart-healthy eating, potentially lowering the risk of cardiovascular diseases, which can impact brain health.

## How to Use This Cookbook

This cookbook is not only a compilation of brain-boosting recipes but also a practical guide to incorporating the Mind Diet into your daily life. Each section offers a diverse selection of recipes designed to make your culinary journey enjoyable and straightforward. Whether you're a seasoned chef or a kitchen novice, we provide step-by-step instructions, nutritional information, and tips to ensure your success.

Our goal is to help you take control of your cognitive health, savor delicious meals, and make the Mind Diet an integral part of your life. As you explore this cookbook, consider it your trusty companion on the path to a brighter, more vibrant future. Your journey to a healthier mind starts right here.

Let's embark on this adventure together, and may every meal be a delightful step toward enhancing your cognitive well-being.

# Chapter 2: The Mind Diet Basics

Welcome to the fundamental chapter of your Mind Diet adventure. In this chapter, we'll go deep into the basic ideas that support the Mind Diet, ensuring that you have a strong understanding of its core concepts before diving into the wonderful dishes that follow.

## What Is the Mind Diet?

The Mind Diet, short for the "Mediterranean-DASH Diet Intervention for Neurodegenerative Delay," is a dietary regimen that has received notice for its ability to maintain cognitive health. It is not a restricted diet but rather a sustainable lifestyle strategy that celebrates particular foods, known as "Mind foods," which have been proven linked to increased brain function and a decreased risk of neurodegenerative illnesses such as

Alzheimer's disease. By adopting the Mind Diet, you are selecting a path that promotes mental clarity, better memory, and general cognitive well-being.

## Key Principles of the Mind Diet

To get the most of the Mind Diet, it's necessary to comprehend its main concepts. These concepts focus around the addition of brain-boosting foods and the elimination of products that might adversely impair cognitive health.

You'll notice that the Mind Diet stresses the following:
- Abundant fruits and veggies
- Whole grains
- Fatty fish - Nuts and seeds
- Olive oil - Lean proteins
- Limited intake of red meat, sweets, and fried foods

These principles offer a dietary framework that not only feeds your brain but also supports your heart health, making it a holistic option for well-rounded vitality.

## Foods to Include and Avoid

In the Mind Diet, some foods are lauded for their extraordinary brain-boosting characteristics. You'll discover a mix of items including leafy greens, berries, nuts, and seafood that take center stage in our meals. On the opposite side, there are products to consume sparingly or avoid completely, such as sweet desserts and processed meals. As you continue through this cookbook, you'll see these recommendations in action, leading you towards delightful meals that enhance your cognitive well-being.

As we explore into the recipes that follow, keep these essential Mind Diet ideas in mind. Embracing this way to eating is more than a food option; it's a lifestyle that supports your mind and body. The trip to a brighter, more vibrant mind begins here in

Chapter 2, establishing the framework for your delightful and wholesome route ahead. Enjoy this chapter, and let's begin out on your Mind Diet trip together!

# Chapter 3: Nutritional Foundations for Brain Health

The things we eat play a key part in supporting brain health and cognitive performance. Optimal diet provides the important building blocks and nutrients necessary for keeping brain health and possibly lowering the risk of cognitive loss.

## Nutrients Essential for Cognitive Function and Brain Health

Several key nutrients are vital for good cognitive function and brain health. These include sugars for energy production, proteins for the creation of hormones, and fats for proper brain structure and communication. Additionally, micronutrients such as vitamins (e.g., B vitamins, vitamin D, vitamin E) and minerals (e.g., iron, zinc, magnesium) are important for various cognitive processes, including memory, information processing, and supporting neural health.

## The Power of Antioxidants in Combating Cognitive Decline

Antioxidants play an important role in fighting oxidative stress, a process that adds to age-related cognitive loss and neurological diseases like Alzheimer's. Antioxidants, such as vitamins C and E, beta-carotene, and other plant substances (polyphenols), help eliminate harmful free radicals in the body, lowering cellular damage, inflammation, and possibly protecting brain cells from harmful oxidative stress.

## Omega-3 Fatty Acids and Their Influence on Brain Health

Omega-3 fatty acids, especially docosahexaenoic acid (DHA), are important for brain health and cognitive performance. DHA is a major component of cell membranes in the brain, and it plays an important part in neural signaling, synapse learning, and inflammation control. Research shows that a proper diet of omega-3 fatty acids may be related with a decreased chance of cognitive loss and better memory.

## Incorporating Vitamins and Minerals for Optimal Cognitive Function

Vitamins and minerals are important for different cognitive processes and keeping general brain health. B vitamins, especially vitamins B6, B12, and folate, are involved in energy production, creation of neurochemicals, and DNA repair processes in the brain. Vitamin D, often referred to as the "sunshine vitamin," has been linked to brain performance and may have a beneficial role. Minerals like iron, zinc, and magnesium are also important for brain processes, neurotransmitter production, and neural health.

## The Importance of Hydration in Supporting Brain Health

Proper water is important for proper brain function. Even slight thirst can affect brain function, attention, and memory. Water plays a vital part in keeping proper blood flow to the brain, clearing out cellular waste products, and ensuring the efficient supply of nutrients and oxygen. Adequate water supports good cognitive function, mental clarity, and general brain health.

Incorporating these food foundations for brain health into our daily meals is key to improving cognitive function and possibly lowering the risk of cognitive decline. Consuming a varied and balanced diet that includes sources of essential nutrients, antioxidants from bright fruits and vegetables, foods rich in omega-3 fatty acids (e.g., fatty fish, flaxseeds), and staying well-hydrated can help to keeping a healthy brain.

While diet is just one part of total brain health, it is an important component when paired with other living factors, such as regular exercise, mental activity, quality sleep, and social interaction. By taking a balanced approach that includes diet and other brain-healthy habits, people can support their cognitive well-being and promote long-term brain health.

# Chapter 4: Foods for Brain Health and Disease Prevention

The foods we consume can greatly impact our brain health and possibly lower the risk of cognitive loss and neurodegenerative illnesses. By adding nutrient-dense foods into our diet, we can feed our brains with important nutrients, vitamins, and healthy fats that support cognitive function and general brain health.

## Exploring Superfoods for Brain Health and Memory Enhancement

Certain foods have gained the reputation of being "superfoods" due to their exceptionally high nutritional value and possible benefits for brain health. Some examples include blueberries, known for their antioxidant qualities and ability to improve memory and brain function. Dark chocolate, rich in flavonoids, may improve blood flow to the brain, memory, and happiness. Other superfoods like ginger, broccoli, and pumpkin seeds are also famous for their brain-boosting potential.

## Brain-Boosting Fruits and veggies Packed with Antioxidants

Fruits and veggies are not only delicious but also provide a wealth of nutrients and antioxidants that support brain health. Berries, such as strawberries, blueberries, and raspberries, are rich in vitamins and have been associated with better memory and brain function. Leafy green veggies like spinach, kale, and Swiss chard are packed with vitamins, minerals, and antioxidants that may lower the chance of cognitive loss. Citrus foods, such as oranges and grapefruits, provide vitamin C, which may have protective effects for the brain.

# Including Healthy Fats and Oils for Optimal Brain Function

Healthy fats and oils are important for optimal brain function, as the brain depends on fats for proper structure and function. Incorporating sources of healthy fats like avocados, nuts, seeds, and fatty fish (e.g., salmon, sardines) can provide omega-3 fatty acids that support brain health and may help lower the chance of cognitive decline. Olive oil, a feature of the Mediterranean diet, is rich in polyunsaturated fats and has been linked with better brain function and a decreased chance of neurological illnesses.

# The Role of Whole Grains and their Impact on Cognitive Health

Whole grains, such as oats, quinoa, brown rice, and whole-wheat bread, provide a steady source of energy to the brain. These complex carbohydrates release glucose slowly, giving a steady stream of food for the brain. Whole grains also add important nutrients like vitamins, minerals, and fiber that support general brain health. Incorporating whole grains into the diet can help keep steady blood sugar levels, improve focus, and support brain function.

## Nourishing Beverages to Support Brain Health

Beverages also offer a chance to feed the brain. Green tea, for example, includes substances that have been shown to improve brain performance and may protect against neurological illnesses. Herbal teas like chamomile and peppermint can have calming effects and promote relaxation, which is helpful for general brain health. Adequate hydration, mainly through water drinking, is important for good brain function and cognitive ability.

By adding these brain-boosting foods and drinks into our daily meals, we can support cognitive function, lower the risk of cognitive loss, and promote good brain health. While individual foods play a part, it's important to accept a varied and healthy diet that includes a wide range of nutrient-dense choices. Pairing a healthy diet with other brain-healthy habits, such as regular exercise, mental activity, quality sleep, and social interaction, can add to general brain health and well-being.

# Chapter 5: 7-Days Mind Diet Meal Planning

**DAY 1:**

**Breakfast: Spinach and Mushroom Omelet with Whole-Grain Toast**

**INGREDIENTS:**

- 3 big eggs
- 1 cup fresh spinach, chopped
- ½ cup mushrooms, sliced
- Salt and pepper to taste
- 1 teaspoon olive oil
- 2 slices of whole-grain bread, toasted

**INSTRUCTIONS:**

1. In a bowl, mix the eggs, salt, and pepper together until well whipped.

2. Heat the olive oil in a non-stick pan over medium heat.

3. Add the mushrooms to the pan and sauté them until they are soft.

4. Add the chopped spinach to the pan and cook for an additional minute until soft.

5. Pour the beaten eggs into the pan, making sure they cover the spinach and mushrooms evenly.

6. Allow the eggs to cook for a few minutes until they start to set.

7. Gently lift the sides of the omelet and tilt the pan to allow the raw eggs to flow to the edges.

8. Once the omelet is mostly set, carefully flip it over to cook the other side quickly.

9. Slide the egg onto a plate and fold it in half.

10. Serve the egg with whole-grain toast on the side and enjoy!

## Lunch: Salmon Salad with Mixed Greens, Avocado, and a Drizzle of Olive Oil

**INGREDIENTS:**

- 4 ounces grilled or baked salmon fillet
- 2 cups mixed veggies
- ½ avocado, sliced
- Cherry tomatoes, split
- Cucumber pieces

- Red onion, thinly sliced
- Lemon pieces (for topping)
- 1 tablespoon extra-virgin olive oil
- Salt and pepper to taste

**INSTRUCTIONS:**
1. In a big bowl, place the mixed veggies.
2. Top the greens with grilled or baked fish, flake it into smaller pieces.
3. Add the chopped avocado, cherry tomatoes, cucumber, and red onion to the bowl.
4. Drizzle the salad with extra-virgin olive oil.
5. Season with salt and pepper to taste.
6. Squeeze fresh lemon juice over the salad for extra taste.
7. Toss gently to mix all the ingredients.
8. Transfer the salad to a plate and serve.

## Dinner: Baked Chicken Breast with Roasted Vegetables and Quinoa

**INGREDIENTS:**
- 4 medium-sized chicken breasts

- 2 cups mixed veggies (such as carrots, bell peppers, zucchini, and broccoli), chopped
- 2 tablespoons olive oil
- 1 teaspoon dried herbs (such as thyme, rosemary, or Italian seasoning)
- Salt and pepper to taste
- 1 cup cooked quinoa

**INSTRUCTIONS:**
1. Preheat the oven to 400°F (200°C).
2. Arrange the chicken breasts on a baking sheet lined with parchment paper.
3. Drizzle the chicken breasts with 1 tablespoon of olive oil and top with dried herbs, salt, and pepper.
4. In a separate bowl, toss the mixed veggies with the leftover olive oil, salt, and pepper.
5. Spread the veggies around the chicken on the baking sheet.
6. Bake in the prepared oven for 20-25 minutes or until the chicken is cooked through and the veggies are soft.

7. While the chicken and veggies are baking, cook the rice according to the package guidelines.

8. Once cooked, fluff the rice with a fork.

9. Serve the baked chicken breast with a side of roasted veggies and rice.

## Snack: Greek Yogurt with Berries and a Sprinkle of Nuts

**INGREDIENTS:**

- ½ cup Greek yogurt
- ½ cup mixed berries (such as blueberries, strawberries, or raspberries)
- 1 tablespoon chopped nuts (such as almonds, walnuts, or pecans)
- Honey (optional, for sweetness)

**INSTRUCTIONS:**

1. In a bowl or serving glass, scoop the Greek yogurt.

2. Top the Greek yogurt with mixed berries.

3. Sprinkle the chopped nuts over the berries.

4. Drizzle the snack with honey if wanted.

5. Mix everything together gently.

6. Enjoy the Greek yogurt with berries and nuts as a healthy snack choice.

## DAY 2:

**Breakfast:  Overnight  Oats  with Flaxseeds, Walnuts, and Cinnamon**

**INGREDIENTS:**

- ½ cup rolled oats
- ½ cup milk (dairy or plant-based)
- 1 tablespoon flaxseeds
- 1 tablespoon chopped walnuts
- ½ teaspoon ground cinnamon
- 1 teaspoon honey or maple syrup (optional, for sweetness)
- Fresh berries for topping (optional)

**INSTRUCTIONS:**

1. In a jar or container, mix the rolled oats, milk, flaxseeds, chopped walnuts, ground cinnamon, and honey or maple syrup (if using).

2. Stir well to mix all the ingredients.

3. Cover the jar or container and chill overnight or for at least 4 hours.

4. In the morning, give the oats a good stir.

5. If wanted, top with fresh berries for extra taste and health benefits.

6. Enjoy the creamy and healthy overnight oats!

## Lunch: Chickpea and Vegetable Stir-Fry with Brown Rice

**INGREDIENTS:**
- 1 cup cooked brown rice
- 1 tablespoon olive oil
- 1 small onion, thinly sliced
- 2 cloves garlic, minced
- 1 red bell pepper, sliced
- 1 zucchini, sliced
- 1 cup broccoli florets
- 1 can (15 ounces) chickpeas, rinsed and drained
- 2 tablespoons low-sodium soy sauce or tamari
- 1 tablespoon rice vinegar
- ½ teaspoon ground ginger

- Salt and pepper to taste

**INSTRUCTIONS:**
1. Heat the olive oil in a big pan or wok over medium-high heat.
2. Add the onion and crushed garlic to the pan and sauté until fragrant and slightly softened.
3. Add the sliced bell pepper, zucchini, and broccoli to the pan. Stir-fry for about 5 minutes or until the veggies are tender-crisp.
4. Add the beans to the pan and cook for an additional 2-3 minutes to heat them through.
5. In a small bowl, mix together the soy sauce or tamari, rice vinegar, ground ginger, salt, and pepper.
6. Pour the sauce over the veggies and beans in the pan. Stir well to coat everything evenly.
7. Serve the stir-fried veggies and beans over a bed of cooked brown rice.

8. Enjoy this delicious and filling lunch choice!

**Dinner: Grilled Turkey Burger Wrapped in Lettuce with Sweet Potato Fries**

**INGREDIENTS:**
- 4 turkey burger patties
- 4 large lettuce leaves (such as romaine or butter lettuce)
- 2 medium-sized sweet potatoes, cut into fries
- 1 tablespoon olive oil
- Salt and pepper to taste
- Optional toppings: cut tomatoes, red onions, avocado, mustard, or any favorite sauces

**INSTRUCTIONS:**
1. Preheat the grill or a grill pan over medium-high heat.
2. Season the turkey burger slices with salt and pepper.

3. Grill the turkey burger patties for about 4-5 minutes per side or until they hit an internal temperature of 165°F (74°C).
4. While the burgers are cooking, warm the oven to 425°F (220°C).
5. Toss the sweet potato fries with olive oil, salt, and pepper on a baking sheet.
6. Spread the fries in a single layer on the baking sheet.
7. Bake the sweet potato fries in the hot oven for about 20-25 minutes, flipping them halfway through until brown and crisp.
8. Once the turkey burger patties are cooked, wrap each piece in a big lettuce leaf.
9. Serve the lettuce-wrapped turkey burgers with a side of crispy sweet potato fries.
10. If wanted, add favorite toppings such as chopped tomatoes, red onions, avocado, or sauces.
11. Enjoy this healthy and low-carb dinner choice!

**INGREDIENTS:**

- ½ cup hummus (store-bought or homemade)
- 1 bell pepper (any color), sliced
- Whole-grain biscuits

**INSTRUCTIONS:**

1. Place the hummus in a bowl or serving dish.

2. Arrange the sliced bell peppers and whole-grain bread on a plate alongside the hummus.

3. Dip the bell pepper slices and bread into the hummus and enjoy this delicious and healthy snack mix!

## DAY 3:



**INGREDIENTS:**

- 1 cup mixed berries (such as blueberries, strawberries, and raspberries)

- ½ cup Greek yogurt
- 1 cup fresh spinach
- 1 tablespoon chia seeds
- ½ cup milk (dairy or plant-based)
- Honey or maple syrup (optional, for sweetness)
- Ice cubes (extra, for preferred thickness)

**INSTRUCTIONS:**

1. In a blender, combine the mixed berries, Greek yogurt, fresh spinach, chia seeds, milk, and a drizzle of honey or maple syrup (if wanted).

2. Blend until smooth and creamy, adding ice cubes if wanted for a thicker consistency.

3. Taste and adjust sweetness if needed by adding more honey or maple syrup.

4. Pour the smoothie into a glass and enjoy the delicious and healthy berry smoothie to start your day.

**INGREDIENTS:**

- 1 cup cooked quinoa
- 1 can (15 ounces) black beans, washed and drained
- 1 cup mixed veggies (such as cherry tomatoes, bell peppers, cucumbers, and red onion), chopped
- Fresh cilantro, chopped
- Juice of 1 lime
- 2 tablespoons extra-virgin olive oil
- Salt and pepper to taste

**INSTRUCTIONS:**

1. In a big bowl, blend the cooked rice, black beans, mixed veggies, and chopped cilantro.
2. In a small bowl, mix together the lime juice, extra-virgin olive oil, salt, and pepper.
3. Pour the sauce over the rice and black bean blend.
4. Toss gently to mix all the ingredients and ensure they are properly coated with the sauce.

5. Taste and fix the spice if needed.

6. Allow the salad to sit for a few minutes to allow the flavors to blend.

7. Serve the quinoa and black bean salad as a refreshing and healthy lunch choice.

## Dinner: Baked Salmon with Steamed Broccoli and Quinoa

**INGREDIENTS:**

- 4 salmon fillets
- 2 tablespoons lemon juice
- 2 tablespoons extra-virgin olive oil
- Salt and pepper to taste
- 2 cups broccoli florets
- 1 cup cooked quinoa
- Fresh dill or parsley for garnish (optional)

**INSTRUCTIONS:**

1. Preheat the oven to 375°F (190°C).

2. Place the salmon pieces on a baking sheet lined with parchment paper.

3. Drizzle the salmon pieces with lemon juice and extra-virgin olive oil.

4. Season the fish with salt and pepper to taste.

5. Bake the salmon in the hot oven for about 12-15 minutes or until it is cooked through and flakes easily with a fork.

6. While the salmon is baking, steam the broccoli pieces until they are tender-crisp.

7. In a serving dish, place the cooked rice, steamed veggies, and baked salmon pieces.

8. Garnish with fresh dill or parsley if wanted.

9. Serve the baked salmon with steamed veggies and rice as a healthy and tasty dinner choice.

## Snack: Apple Slices with Almond Butter

**INGREDIENTS:**

- 1 apple, sliced
- 2 tablespoons almond butter

**INSTRUCTIONS:**

1. Slice the apple into pieces or rounds.

2. Spread the nut butter onto the apple slices.

3. Arrange the apple pieces on a plate.

4. Enjoy the apple pieces with a large layer of almond butter as a tasty and filling snack.

## DAY 4:

### Breakfast: Greek Yogurt Parfait with Mixed Berries and Granola

**INGREDIENTS:**

- 1 cup Greek yogurt
- 1 cup mixed berries (such as blueberries, strawberries, and raspberries)
- ½ cup granola
- Honey or maple syrup (optional, for sweetness)

**INSTRUCTIONS:**

1. In a glass or bowl, add Greek yogurt, mixed berries, and granola.

2. Repeat the stages until the ingredients are used, or change the amounts to your taste.

3. Drizzle with honey or maple syrup if wanted for extra sweetness.

4. Serve the Greek yogurt mixture as a healthy and delicious breakfast choice.

Lunch: Spinach and Feta Stuffed Chicken Breast with Roasted Vegetables

**INGREDIENTS:**
- 4 chicken breast fillets
- 2 cups fresh spinach
- ½ cup crumbled feta cheese
- 1 teaspoon dried oregano
- Salt and pepper to taste
- Olive oil for drizzling
- Assorted veggies for cooking (such as bell peppers, zucchini, and cherry tomatoes)

**INSTRUCTIONS:**
1. Preheat the oven to 400°F (200°C).
2. Using a sharp knife, carefully make a hole into each chicken breast without cutting all the way through.
3. Stuff each chicken breast with fresh spinach and chopped feta cheese.

4. Season the chicken breasts with dried oregano, salt, and pepper.

5. Drizzle with olive oil for extra taste and wetness.

6. Place the stuffed chicken breasts on a baking sheet lined with parchment paper.

7. Arrange the various veggies around the chicken breasts.

8. Roast in the hot oven for about 20-25 minutes, or until the chicken is cooked through and the veggies are soft.

9. Remove from the oven and let it rest for a few minutes.

10. Serve the spinach and feta stuffed chicken breast with roasted vegetables as a healthy and filling lunch choice.

## Dinner: Lentil Curry with Brown Rice

**INGREDIENTS:**
- 1 cup dried beans (any type)
- 1 tablespoon olive oil
- 1 onion, diced
- 2 cloves garlic, chopped
- 1 tablespoon curry powder

- ½ teaspoon ground cumin
- ½ teaspoon ground turmeric
- ½ teaspoon paprika
- 1 can (14 ounces) diced tomatoes
- 1 can (13.5 ounces) coconut milk
- Salt and pepper to taste
- Cooked brown rice for serving
- Fresh cilantro for garnish (optional)

**INSTRUCTIONS:**

1. Cook the beans according to the package guidelines.

2. In a big pan, heat the olive oil over medium heat.

3. Add the chopped onion and crushed garlic to the pan and sauté until fragrant and melted.

4. Stir in the curry powder, ground cumin, ground turmeric, and paprika. Cook for another minute to toast the spices.

5. Add the chopped tomatoes (with their juices) and coconut milk to the pan.

6. Stir well to mix all the ingredients.

7. Bring the mixture to a boil and let it cook for 10 minutes to allow the flavors to meld.

8. Add the cooked lentils to the pan and continue to simmer for an additional 5 minutes.

9. Season with salt and pepper to taste.

10. Serve the lentil sauce over cooked brown rice.

11. Garnish with fresh parsley if wanted.

12. Enjoy the warm and delicious lentil soup with brown rice for a filling dinner.

## Snack: Mixed Nuts and Seeds

**INGREDIENTS:**

- Assorted nuts (such as almonds, walnuts, and peanuts)
- Assorted seeds (such as pumpkin seeds and sunflower seeds)
- Optional: dried cherries or raisins

**INSTRUCTIONS:**

1. In a bowl or airtight container, mix together the various nuts and seeds.

2. Add dried cranberries or raisins if wanted for extra sweetness.

3. Portion out the mixed nuts and seeds into snack-sized pieces or enjoy a bunch as a quick and healthy food.

## DAY 5:

**Breakfast: Vegetable and Goat Cheese Omelet with Whole-Grain Toast**

**INGREDIENTS:**
- 3 big eggs
- ¼ cup mixed veggies (such as bell peppers, onions, and spinach), diced
- ¼ cup chopped goat cheese
- Salt and pepper to taste
- 1 teaspoon olive oil
- 2 slices of whole-grain bread, toasted

**INSTRUCTIONS:**
1. In a bowl, mix the eggs, salt, and pepper together until well whipped.
2. Heat the olive oil in a non-stick pan over medium heat.

3. Add the mixed veggies to the pan and sauté them until they are soft.

4. Pour the beaten eggs into the pan, making sure they cover the veggies evenly.

5. Sprinkle the broken goat cheese on top of the egg.

6. Allow the eggs to cook for a few minutes until they start to set.

7. Gently lift the sides of the omelet and tilt the pan to allow the raw eggs to flow to the edges.

8. Once the omelet is mostly set, carefully flip it over to cook the other side quickly.

9. Slide the egg onto a plate and fold it in half.

10. Serve the omelet with whole-grain toast on the side and enjoy a healthy and full breakfast.

## Lunch: Tuna Salad with Mixed Greens, Tomatoes, and Cucumber

**INGREDIENTS:**

- 1 can (5 ounces) tuna, cleaned
- 2 cups mixed salad greens

- 1 medium-sized tomato, sliced
- ½ cucumber, sliced
- Red onion, thinly sliced
- Lemon pieces (for decoration)
- 1 tablespoon extra-virgin olive oil
- Salt and pepper to taste

**INSTRUCTIONS:**

1. In a bowl, add the drained tuna, mixed salad leaves, tomato slices, cucumber slices, and thinly sliced red onion.

2. Drizzle the salad with extra-virgin olive oil.

3. Season with salt and pepper to taste.

4. Squeeze fresh lemon juice over the salad for extra taste.

5. Toss gently to mix all the ingredients.

6. Transfer the tuna salad to a plate and serve a refreshing and nutritious lunch choice.

## INGREDIENTS:

- 8-10 big shrimp, peeled and deveined
- 1 tablespoon olive oil
- 1 tablespoon fresh lemon juice
- Salt and pepper to taste
- Assorted veggies for grilling (such as bell peppers, zucchini, and cherry tomatoes)
- 1 cup cooked quinoa
- Fresh parsley for garnish (optional)

## INSTRUCTIONS:

1. Preheat the grill or grill pan over medium-high heat.

2. In a bowl, mix the shrimp, olive oil, lemon juice, salt, and pepper. Toss until the shrimp are well covered.

3. Skewer the shrimp onto metal or wet wooden skewers.

4. Grill the shrimp skewers for about 2-3 minutes per side or until they are cooked through and pink.

5. While the shrimp are cooking, brush the various veggies with olive oil and season with salt and pepper.

6. Grill the vegetables until they are soft and slightly brown.

7. Remove the shrimp skewers and cooked veggies from the heat.

8. Serve the grilled shrimp skewers with a side of cooked rice and grilled veggies.

9. Garnish with fresh parsley if wanted.

10. Enjoy a tasty and healthy dinner.

## Snack: Carrot and Celery Sticks with Hummus

**INGREDIENTS:**

- Carrot sticks
- Celery sticks
- Hummus (store-bought or homemade)

**INSTRUCTIONS:**

1. Wash and cut the carrot and celery into sticks.

2. Arrange the carrot and celery sticks on a plate.

3. Serve with a side of hummus for dipping.
4. Enjoy the crunchy and crisp carrot and celery sticks with hummus as a healthy lunch.

## DAY 6:

### Breakfast: Green Smoothie with Kale, Banana, Berries, and Almond Milk

**INGREDIENTS:**
- 1 cup kale leaves, cleaned and ends removed
- 1 ripe banana
- ½ cup mixed berries (such as blueberries, strawberries, and raspberries)
- 1 cup almond milk (or any favorite milk)
- Optional: 1 tablespoon honey or maple syrup for extra sweetness
- Ice cubes (extra, for preferred thickness)

**INSTRUCTIONS:**
1. Place kale, banana, mixed fruit, almond milk, and extra sugar into a mixer.
2. Blend until smooth and creamy. Add ice cubes if needed for a thicker consistency.

3. Taste and adjust sweetness if needed.
4. Pour the green juice into a glass and enjoy a delicious and nutrient-packed meal.

## Lunch: Quinoa and Roasted Vegetable Wrap with a Side Salad

**INGREDIENTS:**

- 1 cup cooked quinoa
- 1 cup roasted veggies (such as bell peppers, zucchini, eggplant, and red onions)
- 1 tablespoon hummus or mayo (optional, for putting on the wrap)
- Large whole-grain wrap or roll
- Mixed salad greens
- Cherry tomatoes, split
- Cucumber pieces
- Dressing of your choice (such as balsamic dressing)

**INSTRUCTIONS:**

1. In a bowl, mix the cooked rice and roasted veggies.
2. Spread hummus or mayo (optional) on the whole-grain wrap.

3. Place a large amount of the rice and roasted veggie filling onto the wrap.

4. Roll the wrap tightly, folding in the sides as you go.

5. In a separate bowl, toss the mixed salad leaves, cherry tomatoes, and cucumber slices with sauce until well covered.

6. Serve the wrap with a side salad and enjoy a full and tasty lunch.

## Dinner: Baked Tofu with Stir-Fried Vegetables and Brown Rice

**INGREDIENTS:**

- 1 block of firm tofu, pressed and cut into cubes
- 2 tablespoons soy sauce or tamari
- 1 tablespoon sesame oil
- 1 tablespoon rice vinegar
- 1 tablespoon honey or maple syrup
- 2 cloves garlic, minced
- 2 cups mixed stir-fry veggies (such as bell peppers, broccoli, carrots, and snap peas)
- Cooked brown rice for serving
- Sesame seeds for garnish (optional)

**INSTRUCTIONS:**

1. Preheat the oven to 400°F (200°C) and line a baking sheet with parchment paper.
2. In a bowl, mix together the soy sauce, sesame oil, rice vinegar, honey or maple syrup, and chopped garlic.
3. Add the tofu cubes to the bowl and toss slowly until well coated in the sauce.
4. Arrange the tofu cubes on the prepared baking sheet.
5. Bake the tofu for 25-30 minutes, or until brown and slightly crisp.
6. While the tofu is baking, heat a pan or wok over medium heat.
7. Add the mixed stir-fry veggies to the pan and stir-fry until tender-crisp.
8. Serve the baked tofu with stir-fried veggies over cooked brown rice.
9. Garnish with sesame seeds if wanted.
10. Enjoy a tasty and healthy dinner.

**INGREDIENTS:**
- ½ cup Greek yogurt
- 1 tablespoon honey (or to taste)
- Sliced nuts for topping

**INSTRUCTIONS:**
1. In a bowl, scoop the Greek yogurt.
2. Drizzle the honey over the Greek yogurt.
3. Sprinkle sliced nuts on top for extra crunch and taste.
4. Mix everything together gently.
5. Enjoy the Greek yogurt with honey and sliced nuts as a filling and protein-rich snack.

**DAY 7:**
**Breakfast: Whole-Grain Toast Topped with Avocado and a Fried Egg**
**INGREDIENTS:**
- 2 slices of whole-grain bread, toasted
- 1 large avocado
- 2 eggs

- Salt and pepper to taste
- Optional toppings: Red pepper powder, chopped parsley, or sliced tomatoes

## INSTRUCTIONS:

1. Smash the avocado in a bowl with a fork until soft.

2. Season with salt and pepper to taste.

3. Spread the chopped avocado evenly onto the toasted whole-grain bread pieces.

4. In a pan, fry the eggs to your chosen doneness (over easy, sunny-side-up, etc.).

5. Gently place one fried egg on top of each avocado-covered toast slice.

6. Optional: Sprinkle with red pepper flakes, chopped parsley, or cut tomatoes for extra flavor and toppings.

7. Enjoy the whole-grain toast topped with avocado and a fried egg for a filling and healthy breakfast.

Lunch: Mediterranean Salad with Mixed Greens, Tomatoes, Cucumbers, Olives, Feta Cheese, and a Drizzle of Olive Oil

## INGREDIENTS:

- 4 cups mixed salad veggies
- 1 cup cherry tomatoes, halved
- 1 cucumber, chopped
- ½ cup kalamata olives, pitted
- ½ cup chopped feta cheese
- Extra-virgin olive oil for drizzling
- Salt and pepper to taste
- Optional: Fresh lemon juice or balsamic vinegar for extra tanginess

## INSTRUCTIONS:

1. In a large bowl, blend the mixed salad leaves, cherry tomatoes, diced cucumber, kalamata olives, and crumbled feta cheese.
2. Drizzle with extra-virgin olive oil and season with salt and pepper to taste.
3. Optional: Squeeze fresh lemon juice or add balsamic vinegar for extra tanginess.

4. Toss gently to mix all the ingredients and ensure they are properly coated with the sauce.

5. Transfer the Mediterranean salad to a plate or separate bowls.

6. Serve quickly as a cool and healthy lunch choice.

**Dinner: Grilled Chicken Breast with Roasted Sweet Potatoes and Green Beans**

**INGREDIENTS:**

- 2 boneless, skinless chicken breast fillets
- 2 medium-sized sweet potatoes, cut into cubes
- 2 cups green beans, cut
- Olive oil for drizzling
- Salt and pepper to taste
- Optional seasonings: Garlic powder, paprika, or dried herbs

**INSTRUCTIONS:**

1. Preheat the grill or grill pan over medium-high heat.

2. Season the chicken breast pieces with salt, pepper, and extra spices of your choice (garlic powder, paprika, or dried herbs).

3. Grill the chicken for about 5-6 minutes per side or until it hits an internal temperature of 165°F (74°C).

4. While the chicken is cooking, warm the oven to 400°F (200°C).

5. On a different baking sheet, toss the sweet potato cubes with olive oil, salt, and pepper.

6. Spread the sweet potato cubes in a single layer on the baking sheet and roast for approximately 20-25 minutes or until they are soft and slightly browned.

7. In the last 10 minutes of cooking the sweet potatoes, add the green beans to the baking sheet. Drizzle with olive oil, salt, and pepper.

8. Continue cooking until the green beans are crisp-tender and lightly brown.

9. Remove the chicken, sweet potatoes, and green beans from heat.

10. Slice the grilled chicken breast pieces.

11. Serve the grilled chicken breast with roasted sweet potatoes and green beans as a healthy and filling dinner choice.



**INGREDIENTS:**
- Assorted fresh fruits (such as berries, melon, pineapple, grapes, and kiwi)
- Optional add-ons: Fresh mint leaves, honey, or a squeeze of lemon juice

**INSTRUCTIONS:**
1. Wash, peel, and chop the fresh fruits into bite-sizcd pieces.
2. In a bowl, mix the various fresh veggies.
3. Optional: Add fresh mint leaves or a squeeze of lemon juice for extra flavor and tanginess.
4. Gently toss to mix all the fruits together.
5. Serve the fresh fruit salad as a light and delicious snack.

*THIS PAGE WAS INTENTIONALLY LEFT BLANK*

# Chapter 6: Alzheimer's Prevention Recipes

A healthy and nutrient-rich diet is important for brain health and lowering the chance of cognitive loss and Alzheimer's disease. By adding delicious and healthy recipes into our daily meals, we can improve our nutrition and support brain energy

## Breakfast Recipes

### 1. Creamy Oatmeal with Berries

**INTRODUCTION:**
Start the day with a cozy bowl of oatmeal filled with brain-boosting vitamins from berries.

**INGREDIENTS:**
- 1/2 cup rolled oats
- 1 cup water or milk of choice
- 1/4 cup mixed berries (blueberries, strawberries, raspberries)

- 1 tablespoon chopped nuts (almonds, walnuts)
- 1 teaspoon honey (optional)

## NUTRITIONAL VALUE:
High in fiber, vitamins, and good fats.

## PREPARATION:
- Cook oats in water or milk until soft.
- Top with berries, nuts, and honey.

## 2. Greek Yogurt Parfait

## INTRODUCTION:
This bright dish mixes probiotic-rich yogurt with fruits and nuts for a healthy and tasty breakfast.

## INGREDIENTS:
- 1/2 cup Greek yogurt
- 1/4 cup granola
- 1/4 cup mixed fruits (banana slices, kiwi, mango)
- 1 tablespoon chopped nuts

**NUTRITIONAL VALUE:**
Good source of protein, bacteria, and vitamins.

**PREPARATION:**
Layer yogurt, granola, fruits, and nuts in a glass.

### 3. Spinach and Mushroom Scramble
**INTRODUCTION:**
A protein-packed scramble with spinach and mushrooms, great for a savory breakfast.

**INGREDIENTS:**
- 2 eggs
- 1/2 cup spinach leaves
- 1/4 cup sliced mushrooms
- 1 tablespoon olive oil
- Salt and pepper to taste

**NUTRITIONAL VALUE:**
Rich in protein, vitamins, and minerals.

**PREPARATION:**
- Sauté mushrooms and spinach in olive oil.
- Add whipped eggs, and mix until cooked.

## 4. Chia Seed Pudding

**INTRODUCTION:**
Make-ahead chia seed pudding loaded with omega-3 fatty acids for brain health.

**INGREDIENTS:**
- 2 tablespoons chia seeds
- 1/2 cup almond milk
- 1/4 teaspoon vanilla flavor
- 1/4 cup diced fruits (berries, banana)

**NUTRITIONAL VALUE:**
High in omega-3s, fiber, and vitamins.

**PREPARATION:**
- Mix chia seeds, almond milk, and vanilla.
- Refrigerate overnight.
- Top with veggies before serving.

## 5. Whole Grain Pancakes

**INTRODUCTION:**

Fluffy whole grain pancakes with a touch of sweetness, great for a hearty breakfast.

**INGREDIENTS:**

- 1/2 cup whole wheat flour
- 1/4 cup oats
- 1 teaspoon baking powder
- 1 egg
- 1/2 cup milk
- 1 tablespoon honey

**NUTRITIONAL VALUE:**

Good source of whole grains and fiber.

**PREPARATION:**

- Mix dry ingredients.
- Add egg, milk, and honey.
- Cook spoonfuls of batter on a pan.

## 6. Veggie Breakfast Burrito

**INTRODUCTION:**

A protein-rich breakfast sandwich packed with bright veggies for a healthy start to the day.

**INGREDIENTS:**

- 1 whole wheat tortilla
- 2 eggs, scrambled
- 1/4 cup black beans
- 2 tablespoons diced bell peppers
- 2 tablespoons diced tomatoes
- 1 tablespoon shredded cheese

**NUTRITIONAL VALUE:**

Provides protein, carbohydrates, and vital nutrients.

**PREPARATION:**

- Fill the tortilla with beaten eggs, beans, veggies, and cheese.
- Roll up and heat.

## 7. Apple Cinnamon Quinoa Bowl

**INTRODUCTION:**

Warm rice mixed with apples and a bit of cinnamon for a healthy and filling breakfast.

**INGREDIENTS:**
- 1/2 cup cooked quinoa
- 1/2 apple, chopped
- 1/4 teaspoon cinnamon
- 1 tablespoon crushed nuts
- 1 teaspoon honey

**NUTRITIONAL VALUE:**

Offers protein, carbohydrates, and vitamins.

**PREPARATION:**
- Mix cooked rice, apple, cinnamon, and nuts.
- Drizzle with honey.

## 8. Peanut Butter Banana Toast

**INTRODUCTION:**

Nutty peanut butter and banana slices on whole grain toast—a quick and easy breakfast pick.

**INGREDIENTS:**

- 1 slice whole grain bread
- 1 tablespoon peanut butter
- 1/2 banana, sliced

**NUTRITIONAL VALUE:**

Provides good fats, potassium, and fiber.

**PREPARATION:**

Spread peanut butter on toast, and top with banana slices.

## 9. Cottage Cheese Fruit Bowl

**INTRODUCTION:**

A relaxing fruit bowl with cottage cheese, giving a mix of energy and vitamins.

**INGREDIENTS:**
- 1/2 cup low-fat cottage cheese
- 1/4 cup mixed fruits (berries, kiwi, pineapple)
- 1 tablespoon sunflower seeds

**NUTRITIONAL VALUE:**
High in protein, calcium, and vitamins.

**PREPARATION:**
Top cottage cheese with veggies and sunflower seeds.

## 10. Blueberry Almond Smoothie

**INTRODUCTION:**
A lovely shake packed with blueberries and nuts for a quick and healthy morning choice.

**INGREDIENTS:**
- 1/2 cup blueberries (fresh or frozen)
- 1/4 cup Greek yogurt
- 1/2 cup almond milk
- 1 tablespoon almond butter
- 1 teaspoon honey

**NUTRITIONAL VALUE:**
Rich in vitamins, protein, and good fats.

**PREPARATION:**
Blend blueberries, yogurt, almond milk, almond butter, and honey until smooth.

Cooking Time: Most meals take around 10-15 minutes to make.

Remember, amount size and food choices should be adjusted to individual nutrition needs and tastes. Enjoy these breakfast choices as part of a healthy Alzheimer's diet.

## Lunch Recipes

### 1. Spinach and Salmon Salad
**INTRODUCTION:**
This salad is rich in omega-3 fatty acids and vitamins, boosting brain health.

**INGREDIENTS:**
- 2 cups baby spinach leaves
- 4 oz grilled salmon, flaked

- 1/4 cup walnuts, chopped
- 1/4 cup blueberries
- 1 tbsp olive oil
- 1 tbsp balsamic vinegar
- Salt and pepper to taste

## PREPARATION:

- Toss spinach, fish, walnuts, and blueberries in a bowl.
- Whisk olive oil, balsamic vinegar, salt, and pepper. Drizzle over the salad.
- Mix gently and serve.

## NUTRITIONAL VALUE:

High in omega-3s, vitamins, and good fats.
Cooking Time: 15 minutes.

## 2. Quinoa and Vegetable Stir-Fry

## INTRODUCTION:

Quinoa is a full protein, while veggies provide important nutrients for brain health.

## INGREDIENTS:

- 1 cup cooked quinoa
- 1 cup mixed veggies (broccoli, bell peppers, carrots)
- 1/4 cup tofu, cubed 2 tsp olive oil
- 2 tsp low-sodium soy sauce
- 1 clove garlic, minced

**PREPARATION:**
- Heat olive oil in a pan.
- Add garlic, tofu, and veggies. Stir-fry for 5 minutes.
- Add cooked rice and soy sauce.
- Cook for an extra 3 minutes.
Serve warm.

**NUTRITIONAL VALUE:**
Protein-rich, filled with fiber, vitamins, and minerals.
Cooking Time: 20 minutes.

## 3. Turkey and Avocado Wrap
**INTRODUCTION:**
This wrap blends lean protein and healthy fats for extended brain energy.

**INGREDIENTS:**
- 1 whole wheat tortilla
3 oz roasted turkey slices
1/2 avocado, sliced
1/4 cup baby spinach leaves
1 tbsp hummus

**PREPARATION:**
- Lay the tortilla flat. Spread hummus on it.
- Layer meat, avocado, and spinach on top.
- Roll up the tortilla and cut in half.

**NUTRITIONAL VALUE:**
Lean protein, good fats, and fiber.
Cooking Time: 10 minutes.

## 4. Lentil and Vegetable Soup

**INTRODUCTION:**
Packed with fiber and plant-based protein, this soup benefits brain function.

**INGREDIENTS:**
- 1 cup cooked green beans

- 1 cup mixed veggies (carrots, celery, zucchini)
- 1/2 onion, chopped 2 cloves garlic, minced
- 4 cups low-sodium veggie soup
- 1 tsp olive oil
- 1/2 tsp turmeric
- Salt and pepper to taste

## PREPARATION:

- Heat olive oil in a pot. Sauté onion and garlic until fragrant.
- Add mixed veggies and cook for 5 minutes.
- Stir in beans, turmeric, salt, and pepper.
- Pour in veggie soup.
- Simmer for 20 minutes.
- Serve hot.

## NUTRITIONAL VALUE:

High in fiber, protein, and vitamins.
Cooking Time: 30 minutes.

## 5. Greek Yogurt Parfait

**INTRODUCTION:**

Greek yogurt offers energy, probiotics, and brain-boosting berries.

**INGREDIENTS:**

- 1 cup plain Greek yogurt
- 1/4 cup mixed berries (blueberries, strawberries)
- 2 tbsp granola
- 1 tsp honey

**PREPARATION:**

- In a glass, add Greek yogurt, berries, and granola.
- Drizzle honey over the top.
- Enjoy as a cool dessert.

**NUTRITIONAL VALUE:**

Protein, bacteria, vitamins, and good fats.
Preparation Time: 5 minutes.

### 6. Sweet Potato and Black Bean Bowl

**INTRODUCTION:**

This bowl is rich in fiber, vitamins, and minerals for brain health.

**INGREDIENTS:**

- 1 medium sweet potato, baked and chopped
- 1/2 cup black beans, drained and rinsed
- 1/4 avocado, sliced 2 tbsp salsa
- 1 tbsp chopped basil
- 1 tsp olive oil

**PREPARATION:**

- Arrange sweet potato, black beans, and avocado in a bowl.
- Drizzle with olive oil and top with salsa and parsley.
- Mix gently and serve.

**NUTRITIONAL VALUE:**

Fiber, vitamins, minerals, and good fats.
Cooking Time: 10 minutes.

## 7. Oatmeal with Almonds and Berries

**INTRODUCTION:**

Oats provide continuous energy, while nuts and berries improve brain health.

**INGREDIENTS:**
- 1/2 cup old-fashioned oats
- 1 cup almond milk
- 1 tbsp nuts, chopped
- 1/4 cup mixed berries
- 1 tsp honey

**PREPARATION:**
- Cook oats in almond milk according to package directions.
- Top with chopped nuts, mixed berries, and a drizzle of honey.
- Enjoy a warm and filling breakfast.

**NUTRITIONAL VALUE:**

Fiber, vitamins, good fats, and steady energy.

Cooking Time: 10 minutes.

## 8. Broccoli and Walnut Stir-Fry

**INTRODUCTION:**

Broccoli and walnuts team up for a nutrient-rich and brain-boosting stir-fry.

**INGREDIENTS:**

- 2 cups broccoli spears
- 1/4 cup walnuts, chopped
- 1/2 cup cooked brown rice
- 1 tbsp olive oil
1 clove garlic, minced
1 tsp low-sodium soy sauce

**PREPARATION:**

- Heat olive oil in a pan. Add garlic and stir-fry for a minute.
- Add broccoli and cook for about 5 minutes until soft.
- Toss in walnuts and cooked brown rice.
- Drizzle with soy sauce, mix well, and serve.

**NUTRITIONAL VALUE:**

Fiber, vitamins, good fats, and vital nutrients.

Cooking Time: 15 minutes.

## 9. Grilled Chicken and Vegetable Skewers

**INTRODUCTION:**

This dish blends lean protein and bright veggies for a well-rounded meal.

**INGREDIENTS:**
- 4 oz grilled chicken breast, cubed
- 1/2 bell pepper, cut into chunks
- 1/2 zucchini, sliced
- 1/2 red onion, cut into chunks
- 1 tsp olive oil
- 1/2 tsp dried herbs (rosemary, thyme)
- Salt and pepper to taste

**PREPARATION:**
- Preheat grill or grill pan.
- Thread chicken, bell pepper, zucchini, and onion onto skewers.
- Brush with olive oil, sprinkle with herbs, salt, and pepper.

- Grill for 10-12 minutes, turning occasionally, until cooked through.
- Serve with a side salad or whole grain.

**NUTRITIONAL VALUE:**
Lean protein, carbohydrates, vitamins, and minerals.
Cooking Time: 20 minutes.

## 10. Berry and Spinach Smoothie
**INTRODUCTION:**
A nutrient-packed drink with berries and veggies to boost brain performance.

**INGREDIENTS:**
- 1 cup fresh spinach leaves
- 1/2 cup mixed berries (strawberries, blueberries, raspberries)
- 1/2 orange
- 1/2 cup unsweetened almond milk
- 1/2 cup water
- 1 tbsp chia seeds

## PREPARATION:
- Blend spinach, mixed berries, banana, almond milk, and water until smooth.
- Add chia seeds and mix for a few seconds.
- Pour into a glass and enjoy the cool drink.

## NUTRITIONAL VALUE:
Antioxidants, vitamins, minerals, fiber, and good fats.
Preparation Time: 5 minutes.

## Dinner Recipes

### 1. Baked Salmon with Quinoa:
## INTRODUCTION:
A brain-boosting dinner rich in omega-3 fatty acids and protein.

## INGREDIENTS:
- 2 salmon pieces
- 1 cup quinoa
- 2 cups low-sodium chicken broth
- 1 cup broccoli sprouts
- 1 lemon
- Olive oil, salt, and pepper

**NUTRITIONAL VALUE:**
High in protein, omega-3s, and carbohydrates.
Cooking Time: 30 minutes.

**PREPARATION:**
- Preheat oven to 375°F (190°C).
- Season salmon with olive oil, salt, pepper, and lemon juice.
- Bake salmon for 15-20 minutes.
- Cook rice in chicken soup.
- Steam veggies and serve alongside salmon and rice.

## 2. Mediterranean Chickpea Salad:

**INTRODUCTION:**
A bright salad packed with vitamins and good fats.

**INGREDIENTS:**
- 1 can chickpeas, washed
- 1 cucumber, diced 1 cup cherry tomatoes, half

- 1/4 cup red onion, finely chopped
- 1/4 cup feta cheese, crumbled
- 2 tbsp olive oil
- 1 tbsp balsamic vinegar
- Fresh herbs (e.g., parsley, basil)

**NUTRITIONAL VALUE:**
Rich in fiber, vitamins, and good fats.
Cooking Time: 15 minutes.

**PREPARATION:**
- Mix beans, cucumber, tomatoes, red onion, and feta.
- Whisk olive oil, balsamic vinegar, and herbs for sauce.
- Toss salad with dressing before serving.

## 3. Stir-Fried Tofu and Vegetables:
**INTRODUCTION:**
A plant-based stir-fry for a healthy meal.
**INGREDIENTS:**
- 8 oz tofu, cubed
- 2 cups mixed veggies (bell peppers, broccoli, carrots)

- 2 cloves garlic, minced
- 2 tbsp low-sodium soy sauce
- 1 tbsp sesame oil
- 1 tsp ginger, grated

**NUTRITIONAL VALUE:**
Provides protein, carbohydrates, and vital nutrients.
Cooking Time: 20 minutes.

**PREPARATION:**
- Sauté tofu in sesame oil until brown.
- Add garlic, ginger, and veggies.
- Stir in soy sauce and cook until veggies are soft.

## 4. Roasted Chicken with Sweet Potatoes:

**INTRODUCTION:**
A filling meal with lean protein and complicated carbs.

**INGREDIENTS:**
- 2 boneless, skinless chicken breasts

- 2 sweet potatoes, peeled and chopped
- 1 tbsp olive oil
- 1 tsp rosemary, chopped
- Salt and pepper

**NUTRITIONAL VALUE:**
Rich in protein, vitamin A, and potassium.
Cooking Time: 40 minutes.

**PREPARATION:**
- Season chicken with rosemary, salt, and pepper.
- Toss sweet potatoes with olive oil, salt, and pepper.
- Roast chicken and sweet potatoes in the oven at 400°F (200°C) for 25-30 minutes.

## 5. Spinach and Mushroom Omelette:
**INTRODUCTION:**
A nutrient-dense egg for a quick dinner.

**INGREDIENTS:**
- 3 eggs
- 1 cup spinach, chopped

- 1/2 cup mushrooms, chopped
- 1/4 cup low-fat cheese, grated
- Cooking spray or olive oil
- Salt and pepper

**NUTRITIONAL VALUE:**
High in protein, vitamins, and minerals.
Cooking Time: 15 minutes.

**PREPARATION:**
- Sauté mushrooms and spinach until soft.
- Whisk eggs and season with salt and pepper.
- Pour eggs into the pan, add cheese, and cook until set.

## 6. Lentil and Vegetable Stew:

**INTRODUCTION:**
A warming stew filled with plant-based energy and fiber.

**INGREDIENTS:**
- 1 cup green beans
- 2 carrots, diced

- 2 celery stalks, diced 1 onion, chopped 3 cloves garlic, minced
- 4 cups low-sodium veggie soup
- 1 tsp thyme
- Salt and pepper

**NUTRITIONAL VALUE:**
High in protein, fiber, and vital nutrients.
Cooking Time: 45 minutes.

**PREPARATION:**
- Sauté onion, garlic, carrots, and celery.
- Add beans, thyme, and veggie broth.
- Simmer until lentils are tender.

## 7. Grilled Turkey Burgers with Avocado:

**INTRODUCTION:**
Lean turkey burgers mixed with brain-healthy avocado.

**INGREDIENTS:**
- 1 lb chopped turkey
- 1 avocado, sliced

- Whole wheat burger buns
- Lettuce, tomato, onion (optional)
- Salt, pepper, and herbs (e.g., oregano, basil)

**NUTRITIONAL VALUE:**
Low-fat protein and good fats.
Cooking Time: 20 minutes.

**PREPARATION:**
- Mix ground turkey with herbs, salt, and pepper.
- Shape into patties and cook for about 5-6 minutes on each side.
- Assemble burgers with avocado slices and extra toppings.

## 8. Quinoa and Vegetable Stir-Fry:

**INTRODUCTION:**
A adaptable stir-fry with protein-packed quinoa.

**INGREDIENTS:**
- 1 cup quinoa

- 2 cups mixed veggies (peas, bell peppers, carrots)
- 2 green onions, chopped
- 2 tbsp low-sodium soy sauce
- 1 tbsp olive oil
- 1 tsp garlic, minced

## NUTRITIONAL VALUE:
Protein, carbohydrates, and a range of vitamins.
Cooking Time: 25 minutes.

## PREPARATION:
- Cook quinoa according to package directions.
- Sauté veggies in olive oil and garlic.
- Stir in cooked rice and soy sauce.

9. Baked Cod with Steamed Vegetables:

## INTRODUCTION:
Light and crispy baked cod with a side of veggies.

Ingredients:
- 2 cod pieces
- 2 cups mixed veggies (zucchini, carrots, cabbage)
- Lemon zest and juice
- Fresh dill (optional)
- Salt, pepper, and olive oil

**NUTRITIONAL VALUE:**
Lean protein and vitamins.
Cooking Time: 25 minutes.

**PREPARATION:**
- Season cod with lemon juice, salt, and pepper.
- Bake cod in the oven at 350°F (175°C) for 15-20 minutes.
- Steam veggies and drizzle with olive oil and lemon juice.

## 10. Vegetable and Bean Stir-Fry:
**INTRODUCTION:**
A fiber-rich stir-fry featuring beans and bright veggies.

**INGREDIENTS:**
- 1 can mixed beans, drained and rinsed
- 2 cups mixed veggies (snap peas, bell peppers, broccoli)
- 2 tbsp low-sodium teriyaki sauce
- 1 tbsp sesame oil
- 1 tsp sesame seeds

**NUTRITIONAL VALUE:**
Protein, fiber, and a range of vitamins.
Cooking Time: 20 minutes.
**PREPARATION:**
- Sauté mixed veggies in scsame oil.
- Add beans and teriyaki sauce, stir-fry for a few minutes.
- Garnish with sesame seeds before serving.

Enjoy thcsc healthy Alzheimer's diet dinner recipes made to support brain health!

## 1. Blueberry-almond Parfait:

**INTRODUCTION:**
This antioxidant-rich snack helps support brain health with the goodness of blueberries and almonds.

**INGREDIENTS:**
- 1/2 cup Greek yogurt
- 1/4 cup blueberries
- 1 tablespoon chopped nuts
- 1 teaspoon honey

**PREPARATION:**
- Layer yogurt, blueberries, and chopped nuts in a glass.
- Drizzle honey on top. Enjoy immediately.

**NUTRITIONAL VALUE:**
Approx. 180 calories, 8g protein, 15g carbs, 10g fat.
Cooking Time: 5 minutes.

## INTRODUCTION:

Packed with healthy fats and omega-3s, this snack is a great way to feed the brain.

## INGREDIENTS:

- 1 slice whole grain bread
- 1/2 avocado, mashed
- 2 oz smoked salmon
- 1 teaspoon lemon juice

## PREPARATION:

- Toast the bread. Spread mashed avocado on top.
- Place smoked salmon and drizzle with lemon juice.

## NUTRITIONAL VALUE:

Approx. 250 calories, 15g protein, 20g carbs, 13g fat.
Cooking Time: 10 minutes.

**3. Spinach and Feta Stuffed Mushrooms:**

## INTRODUCTION:

These stuffed mushrooms provide a dose of vitamin K and antioxidants from spinach.

Ingredients:
- 6 large mushrooms
- 1 cup baby spinach, chopped
- 1/4 cup crumbled feta cheese
- 1 tablespoon olive oil

## PREPARATION:

- Remove mushroom branches. Sauté spinach with olive oil.
- Fill mushrooms with spinach and feta combination.
- Bake at 350°F for 15 minutes.

## NUTRITIONAL VALUE:

Approx. 90 calories, 5g protein, 4g carbs, 6g fat.

Cooking Time: 25 minutes.

## 4. Trail Mix with Nuts and Berries:

**INTRODUCTION:**

A nutrient-packed snack mixing nuts and berries to provide important vitamins and healthy fats.

**INGREDIENTS:**

- 1/4 cup mixed nuts (almonds, walnuts, cashews)
- 2 tablespoons dried cranberries
- 2 tablespoons dark chocolate chips

**PREPARATION:**

- Mix all items in a bowl.
- Portion into snack-sized bags for ease.

**NUTRITIONAL VALUE:**

Approx. 200 calories, 5g protein, 15g carbs, 14g fat.
Cooking Time: 5 minutes.

## 5. Cucumber And Hummus Slices:

**INTRODUCTION:**

This cool snack pairs hydrating cucumbers with protein-packed hummus.

**INGREDIENTS:**

- 1 medium cucumber, chopped
- 1/4 cup hummus

**PREPARATION:**

- Arrange cucumber pieces on a plate.
- Serve with a side of hummus for dipping.

**NUTRITIONAL VALUE:**

Approx. 100 calories, 4g protein, 10g carbs, 6g fat.
Cooking Time: 5 minutes.

## 6. Quinoa Fruit Salad:

**INTRODUCTION:**

A nutrient-dense fruit salad with rice for prolonged energy and vitamins.

**INGREDIENTS:**
- 1/2 cup cooked quinoa
- 1/2 cup mixed fruits (berries, mango, kiwi)
- 2 tablespoons chopped nuts (pistachios, almonds)
- 1 teaspoon honey

**PREPARATION:**
- Combine cooked rice, mixed veggies, and chopped nuts.
- Drizzle with honey and toss gently.

**NUTRITIONAL VALUE:**
Approx. 220 calories, 5g protein, 35g carbs, 7g fat.
Cooking Time: 15 minutes.

## 7. Cottage Cheese with Berries:

**INTRODUCTION:**
Protein-rich cottage cheese mixed with antioxidant-loaded berries makes for a filling snack.

**INGREDIENTS:**
- 1/2 cup low-fat cottage cheese
- 1/4 cup mixed berries (blueberries, strawberries)
- 1 teaspoon chia seeds

**PREPARATION:**
- Top cottage cheese with mixed veggies and chia seeds.

**NUTRITIONAL VALUE:**
Approx. 150 calories, 15g protein, 15g carbs, 4g fat.
Cooking Time: 5 minutes.

## 8. Dark Chocolate-Dipped Banana Bites:

**INTRODUCTION:**
A sweet treat with dark chocolate and bananas, giving vitamins and potassium.

**INGREDIENTS:**
- 1 ripe banana, cut into bite-sized pieces
- 2 oz dark chocolate, melted

- 1 tablespoon chopped nuts (walnuts, almonds)

**PREPARATION:**
- Dip banana pieces in melted dark chocolate, then sprinkle with chopped nuts.
- Place on parchment paper and let the chocolate set.

**NUTRITIONAL VALUE:**
Approx. 160 calories, 2g protein, 20g carbs, 9g fat.
Cooking Time: 20 minutes (including chocolate setting time).

## 9. Roasted Chickpeas:
**INTRODUCTION:**
A crunchy snack packed with fiber and protein from roasted chickpeas.

**INGREDIENTS:**
- 1 can (15 oz) chickpeas, drained and washed
- 1 tablespoon olive oil

- 1 teaspoon crushed cumin
- 1/2 teaspoon paprika
- Salt to taste

**PREPARATION:**
- Toss beans with olive oil and spices.
- Roast at 400°F for 20-25 minutes, until crispy.

**NUTRITIONAL VALUE:**
Approx. 150 calories, 6g protein, 22g carbs, 4g fat.
Cooking Time: 30 minutes.

## 10. Veggie and Cheese Quesadilla:
**INTRODUCTION:**
A tasty snack filled with veggies and cheese, giving a mix of nutrients.

**INGREDIENTS:**
- 1 whole wheat tortilla
- 1/4 cup shredded cheese (cheddar, mozzarella)

- 1/4 cup mixed chopped veggies (bell peppers, onions, tomatoes)
- 1 teaspoon olive oil

## PREPARATION:

- Sauté cut veggies in olive oil.
- Place half of the chopped cheese on one side of the tortilla, top with sautéed veggies, and leftover cheese.
- Fold tortilla in half and cook on a pan until cheese melts and tortilla is crispy.

## NUTRITIONAL VALUE:

Approx. 250 calories, 10g protein, 30g carbs, 10g fat.
Cooking Time: 15 minutes.

Enjoy these wonderful snacks while supporting your body and brain.

# Dessert Recipes

**1. Blueberry Oatmeal Bars:**

**INTRODUCTION:**

These bars are packed with vitamins from blueberries and fiber from oats, great for a brain-healthy snack.

**INGREDIENTS:**

- 2 cups rolled oats
- 1 cup whole wheat flour
- 1/2 cup coconut oil
- 1/4 cup honey
- 1 cup fresh blueberries

**PREPARATION:**

- Preheat oven to 350°F (175°C).
- Mix oats, flour, coconut oil, and honey to make a thick mixture.
- Press 2/3 of the butter into a baking pan.
- Spread strawberries over the crust.
- Sprinkle leftover oat mixture on top.
- Bake for 25-30 minutes.

**NUTRITIONAL VALUE:**
High in fiber and vitamins.
Cooking Time: 25-30 minutes.

## 2. Chia Pudding:
**INTRODUCTION:**
Chia seeds are rich in Omega-3 fatty acids and fiber, making this pudding a great dessert choice.

**INGREDIENTS:**
- 1/4 cup chia seeds
- 1 cup almond milk
- 1 tbsp honey
- 1/2 tsp vanilla flavor

**PREPARATION:**
- Mix chia seeds, almond milk, honey, and vanilla extract.
- Stir well, then chill for a few hours or overnight.
- Serve topped with fresh berries.

**NUTRITIONAL VALUE:**
Omega-3s and fiber-rich.
Cooking Time: 5 minutes (plus cooling time).

### 3. Banana Ice Cream:
Introduction:
A simple and healthy frozen treat using just one ingredient – bananas.

**INGREDIENTS:**
- 4 ripe bananas, sliced and frozen

**PREPARATION:**
- Blend frozen banana slices in a food processor until creamy.
Serve directly as soft-serve or freeze for firmer consistency.

**NUTRITIONAL VALUE:**
Natural carbs and potassium.
Cooking Time: 5 minutes.

## INTRODUCTION:

Warm, cinnamon-spiced baked apples are a cozy dessert choice that's gentle on the senses.

## INGREDIENTS:

- 4 apples, cored
- 2 tbsp chopped nuts (walnuts, almonds)
- 2 tbsp raisins
- 1 tsp cinnamon

## PREPARATION:

- Preheat oven to 375°F (190°C).
- Mix nuts, raisins, and cinnamon.
- Stuff the cored apples with the mixture.
- Place apples in a baking dish and add a bit of water.
- Bake for 25-30 minutes.

## NUTRITIONAL VALUE:

Rich in fiber and vitamins.
Cooking Time: 25-30 minutes.

## INTRODUCTION:

Creamy Greek yogurt piled with fruits and nuts offers a balanced and nutrient-rich snack.

## INGREDIENTS:

- 1 cup Greek yogurt
- 1/2 cup mixed berries (blueberries, strawberries)
- 2 tbsp chopped almonds
- 1 tsp honey

## PREPARATION:

- In a glass, add Greek yogurt, mixed berries, and chopped nuts.
- Drizzle honey on top.

## NUTRITIONAL VALUE:

Protein, vitamins, and antioxidants.
Cooking Time: 5 minutes.

## INTRODUCTION:

This pumpkin-flavored treat is high in Omega-3s and gives a boost of vitamins and minerals.

## INGREDIENTS:

- 1/2 cup pumpkin puree
- 2 tbsp chia seeds
- 1/2 tsp pumpkin pie spice
- 1 tbsp maple syrup

## PREPARATION:

- Mix pumpkin juice, chia seeds, pumpkin pie spice, and maple syrup.
- Refrigerate for a few hours or overnight.

## NUTRITIONAL VALUE:

Omega-3s, vitamins, and fiber.
Cooking Time: 5 minutes (plus cooling time).

## 7. Cocoa Avocado Pudding:

**INTRODUCTION:**
Creamy avocado-based pudding with cocoa is a delicious sweet that's also loaded with healthy fats.

**INGREDIENTS:**
- 2 ripe avocados
- 1/4 cup unsweetened cocoa powder
- 1/4 cup honey
- 1 tsp vanilla flavor

**PREPARATION:**
- Blend avocados, chocolate powder, honey, and vanilla extract until smooth.
- Refrigerate for at least 1 hour before serving.

**NUTRITIONAL VALUE:**
Healthy fats and vitamins.
Cooking Time: 10 minutes (plus cooling time).

## 8. Berry Sorbet:

## INTRODUCTION:

A refreshing dessert made from mixed berries, giving a burst of vitamins and natural sweetness.

## INGREDIENTS:

- 2 cups mixed berries (raspberries, blackberries, strawberries)
- 1/4 cup honey
- 1 tbsp lemon juice

## PREPARATION:

- Blend berries, honcy, and lemon juice until smooth.
- Pour mixture into a small dish and freeze for 2-3 hours, shaking every 30 minutes.

## NUTRITIONAL VALUE:

Antioxidants and vitamins.
Cooking Time: 10 minutes (plus cooling time).

## 9. Coconut Rice Pudding:

### INTRODUCTION:

Creamy coconut rice pudding is a cozy dessert choice that's easy to digest.

### INGREDIENTS:

- 1/2 cup Arborio rice
- 1 can (13.5 oz) coconut milk
- 2 tbsp honey
- 1/2 tsp vanilla flavor

### PREPARATION:

- Cook rice in coconut milk until soft.
- Stir in honey and vanilla extract.
- Simmer until mixture thickens.

### NUTRITIONAL VALUE:

Healthy fats and ease.
Cooking Time: 30 minutes.

## 10. Almond Butter Bites:

### INTRODUCTION:

Nutty nut butter bites are a filling snack filled with protein and healthy fats.

## INGREDIENTS:
- 1 cup almond butter
- 1/4 cup honey
- 1 cup rolled oats
- 1/2 cup crushed dark chocolate

## PREPARATION:
- Mix almond butter, honey, oats, and chopped chocolate.
- Shape into bite-sized balls and chill for 1 hour.

## NUTRITIONAL VALUE:
Protein and good fats.
Cooking Time: 10 minutes (plus cooling time).

*THIS PAGE WAS INTENTIONALLY LEFT BLANK*

# Conclusion

In summary, the "Mind Diet Cookbook for Seniors" is your recipe for a healthier, more robust mind. It's not simply a compilation of great recipes; it's a trip into cognitive vigor. As you've studied these pages, you've found the extraordinary potential of "Mind foods," the culinary treasures that may increase your memory and brain function.

But this isn't just about meals; it's a commitment to your emotional well-being. Your journey to a sharper, more nimble mind is as easy as accepting the concepts inside this cookbook. With every mouthful, you're nourishing your cognitive wellness.

So, make this cookbook your constant friend, your gastronomic guide to greater brain health. Use it to relish every taste life has to offer while nourishing your most important asset: your intellect. Let this conclusion be a call to action, a reminder that a brighter, more vivid intellect is definitely within your grasp. The road to cognitive vigor starts here.

# Contact Us

Dear valued reader,

First and foremost, I would like to express my sincere gratitude for choosing my book **MIND DIET COOKBOOK FOR SENIORS** as your guide. I hope that you found the content helpful, informative, and enjoyable to read.

As a valued customer, I would like to offer you an exclusive bonus - a free **SPECIAL MEAL TRACKER** and you will find it in the next page.

I also want to remind you that your review/feedback is important to me. I would love to hear your thoughts, observations, questions and suggestions about the book, so that I can continue to improve and provide you with even more valuable content in the future.

You can contact me through this email:
Coreyhelpdesk@gmail.com

Thank you once again for choosing my book, and I look forward to hearing from you soon!

Best regards,
Corey Pearce

# BONUS - SPECIAL MEAL TRACKER

## SPECIAL MEAL TRACKER

DATE:..............................

| | | |
|---|---|---|
| **MONDAY** | BREAKFAST | |
| | LUNCH | |
| | DINNER | |
| **TUESDAY** | BREAKFAST | |
| | LUNCH | |
| | DINNER | |
| **WEDNESDAY** | BREAKFAST | |
| | LUNCH | |
| | DINNER | |
| **THURSDAY** | BREAKFAST | |
| | LUNCH | |
| | DINNER | |
| **FRIDAY** | BREAKFAST | |
| | LUNCH | |
| | DINNER | |
| **SATURDAY** | BREAKFAST | |
| | LUNCH | |
| | DINNER | |
| **SUNDAY** | BREAKFAST | |
| | LUNCH | |
| | DINNER | |

| SNACKS |
|---|
| |

| NOTE |
|---|
| |

# SPECIAL MEAL TRACKER

DATE:................................

| | | |
|---|---|---|
| **MONDAY** | BREAKFAST | |
| | LUNCH | |
| | DINNER | |
| **TUESDAY** | BREAKFAST | |
| | LUNCH | |
| | DINNER | |
| **WEDNESDAY** | BREAKFAST | |
| | LUNCH | |
| | DINNER | |
| **THURSDAY** | BREAKFAST | |
| | LUNCH | |
| | DINNER | |
| **FRIDAY** | BREAKFAST | |
| | LUNCH | |
| | DINNER | |
| **SATURDAY** | BREAKFAST | |
| | LUNCH | |
| | DINNER | |
| **SUNDAY** | BREAKFAST | |
| | LUNCH | |
| | DINNER | |

**SNACKS**

**NOTE**

# SPECIAL MEAL TRACKER

DATE:................................

| | | |
|---|---|---|
| **MONDAY** | BREAKFAST | |
| | LUNCH | |
| | DINNER | |
| **TUESDAY** | BREAKFAST | |
| | LUNCH | |
| | DINNER | |
| **WEDNESDAY** | BREAKFAST | |
| | LUNCH | |
| | DINNER | |
| **THURSDAY** | BREAKFAST | |
| | LUNCH | |
| | DINNER | |
| **FRIDAY** | BREAKFAST | |
| | LUNCH | |
| | DINNER | |
| **SATURDAY** | BREAKFAST | |
| | LUNCH | |
| | DINNER | |
| **SUNDAY** | BREAKFAST | |
| | LUNCH | |
| | DINNER | |

SNACKS

NOTE

# SPECIAL MEAL TRACKER

DATE:.................................

| | | |
|---|---|---|
| **MONDAY** | BREAKFAST | |
| | LUNCH | |
| | DINNER | |
| **TUESDAY** | BREAKFAST | |
| | LUNCH | |
| | DINNER | |
| **WEDNESDAY** | BREAKFAST | |
| | LUNCH | |
| | DINNER | |
| **THURSDAY** | BREAKFAST | |
| | LUNCH | |
| | DINNER | |
| **FRIDAY** | BREAKFAST | |
| | LUNCH | |
| | DINNER | |
| **SATURDAY** | BREAKFAST | |
| | LUNCH | |
| | DINNER | |
| **SUNDAY** | BREAKFAST | |
| | LUNCH | |
| | DINNER | |

SNACKS

NOTE

# SPECIAL MEAL TRACKER

DATE:.................................

| | | |
|---|---|---|
| **MONDAY** | BREAKFAST | |
| | LUNCH | |
| | DINNER | |
| **TUESDAY** | BREAKFAST | |
| | LUNCH | |
| | DINNER | |
| **WEDNESDAY** | BREAKFAST | |
| | LUNCH | |
| | DINNER | |
| **THURSDAY** | BREAKFAST | |
| | LUNCH | |
| | DINNER | |
| **FRIDAY** | BREAKFAST | |
| | LUNCH | |
| | DINNER | |
| **SATURDAY** | BREAKFAST | |
| | LUNCH | |
| | DINNER | |
| **SUNDAY** | BREAKFAST | |
| | LUNCH | |
| | DINNER | |

SNACKS

NOTE

# SPECIAL MEAL TRACKER

DATE:.................................

| | | | SNACKS |
|---|---|---|---|
| **MONDAY** | BREAKFAST | | |
| | LUNCH | | |
| | DINNER | | |
| **TUESDAY** | BREAKFAST | | |
| | LUNCH | | |
| | DINNER | | |
| **WEDNESDAY** | BREAKFAST | | |
| | LUNCH | | |
| | DINNER | | |
| **THURSDAY** | BREAKFAST | | |
| | LUNCH | | |
| | DINNER | | |
| **FRIDAY** | BREAKFAST | | NOTE |
| | LUNCH | | |
| | DINNER | | |
| **SATURDAY** | BREAKFAST | | |
| | LUNCH | | |
| | DINNER | | |
| **SUNDAY** | BREAKFAST | | |
| | LUNCH | | |
| | DINNER | | |

# SPECIAL MEAL TRACKER

**DATE:**.................................

| | | | SNACKS |
|---|---|---|---|
| **MONDAY** | BREAKFAST | | |
| | LUNCH | | |
| | DINNER | | |
| **TUESDAY** | BREAKFAST | | |
| | LUNCH | | |
| | DINNER | | |
| **WEDNESDAY** | BREAKFAST | | |
| | LUNCH | | |
| | DINNER | | |
| **THURSDAY** | BREAKFAST | | |
| | LUNCH | | |
| | DINNER | | |
| **FRIDAY** | BREAKFAST | | |
| | LUNCH | | NOTE |
| | DINNER | | |
| **SATURDAY** | BREAKFAST | | |
| | LUNCH | | |
| | DINNER | | |
| **SUNDAY** | BREAKFAST | | |
| | LUNCH | | |
| | DINNER | | |

# SPECIAL MEAL TRACKER

**DATE:**......................................

| | | | SNACKS |
|---|---|---|---|
| **MONDAY** | BREAKFAST | | |
| | LUNCH | | |
| | DINNER | | |
| **TUESDAY** | BREAKFAST | | |
| | LUNCH | | |
| | DINNER | | |
| **WEDNESDAY** | BREAKFAST | | |
| | LUNCH | | |
| | DINNER | | |
| **THURSDAY** | BREAKFAST | | |
| | LUNCH | | |
| | DINNER | | |
| **FRIDAY** | BREAKFAST | | NOTE |
| | LUNCH | | |
| | DINNER | | |
| **SATURDAY** | BREAKFAST | | |
| | LUNCH | | |
| | DINNER | | |
| **SUNDAY** | BREAKFAST | | |
| | LUNCH | | |
| | DINNER | | |

# SPECIAL MEAL TRACKER

DATE:..................................

| | | |
|---|---|---|
| **MONDAY** | BREAKFAST | |
| | LUNCH | |
| | DINNER | |
| **TUESDAY** | BREAKFAST | |
| | LUNCH | |
| | DINNER | |
| **WEDNESDAY** | BREAKFAST | |
| | LUNCH | |
| | DINNER | |
| **THURSDAY** | BREAKFAST | |
| | LUNCH | |
| | DINNER | |
| **FRIDAY** | BREAKFAST | |
| | LUNCH | |
| | DINNER | |
| **SATURDAY** | BREAKFAST | |
| | LUNCH | |
| | DINNER | |
| **SUNDAY** | BREAKFAST | |
| | LUNCH | |
| | DINNER | |

| SNACKS |
|---|
| |

| NOTE |
|---|
| |

# SPECIAL MEAL TRACKER

DATE:........................................

| | | | SNACKS |
|---|---|---|---|
| **MONDAY** | BREAKFAST | | |
| | LUNCH | | |
| | DINNER | | |
| **TUESDAY** | BREAKFAST | | |
| | LUNCH | | |
| | DINNER | | |
| **WEDNESDAY** | BREAKFAST | | |
| | LUNCH | | |
| | DINNER | | |
| **THURSDAY** | BREAKFAST | | |
| | LUNCH | | |
| | DINNER | | |
| **FRIDAY** | BREAKFAST | | NOTE |
| | LUNCH | | |
| | DINNER | | |
| **SATURDAY** | BREAKFAST | | |
| | LUNCH | | |
| | DINNER | | |
| **SUNDAY** | BREAKFAST | | |
| | LUNCH | | |
| | DINNER | | |